The Big Nap

How We Failed to Forsee History's Pandemics, From Bubonic Plague to The Spanish Flu of 1918 to Right Now!

James Simon

contained within this document, including, but not limited to, errors, omissions, or inaccuracies.

Table of Contents

Introduction

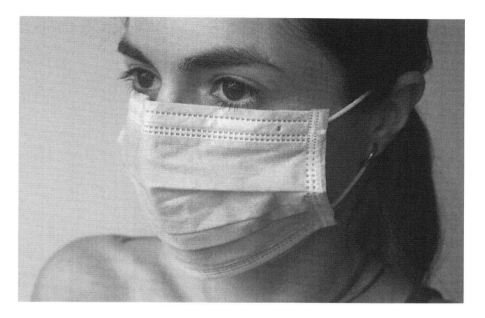

Face Mask

Evolution is why the human race has been able to assert itself as the dominant living species in all of the world. In spite of the many threats and dangers that our species has been confronted with, we have always managed to find a way to persevere. No one has been able to rationalize the idea of human relentlessness more eloquently than Charles Darwin when he introduced to the world the Theory of Evolution by Natural Selection.

To put it simply, Darwin asserted that if anyone or anything is to survive in this world, it must learn to adapt. This is exactly what the human species has been able to do all throughout its history. Since the earliest civilizations, human beings have been continually finding ways to make their lives easier and more convenient by developing new technologies. Sometimes, this technology came in the form of material objects like weapons, clothes, tools, housing structures, and motor vehicles. At other times, this technology came in the form of social structures like governments, communities, charitable institutions, and academic institutions. Through the development of these technologies, the human race has proven its ability to adapt to an ever changing and unforgiving world. By developing itself on a gradual and consistent basis, the human race has been able to arm itself against the various threats that it has faced throughout the years.

Imagine any threat that could potentially push our species to complete extinction. Maybe a large enough meteor will eventually find its way into earth's gravitational pull and annihilate all existence as we know it. The land that we stand on could cave in on itself and swallow all of us whole. Maybe something like global warming will eventually reach levels that could spell disaster for us. Sure, some of the ideas that you come up with may be possible and some may not. However, there is one particular threat that you should never discount when it comes to ending human civilization as we know it: a pandemic.

What is a Pandemic?

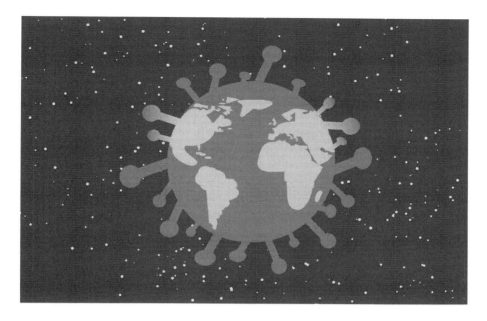

Viral Outbreak

Before diving into the fine details of pandemics, it might be best to explore the technicalities and definitions behind pandemics and what they really mean. You might already know that a pandemic stems from the uncontrolled spread of an infectious disease. However, not all of these diseases are created equally. You might be familiar with phrases like outbreaks, pandemics, and epidemics, but you might not really know what the distinctions are.

These are generally just classifications that the scientific and medical community attributes to certain diseases depending on how strong and infectious they are. A lot of people tend to interchange these words when engaged in informal or casual conversations. However, for the sake of clarity and precision, it would be best to really understand the nuances behind each classification. Once you gain a better grasp and understanding of these words, you are in a better position to understand emerging news surrounding public health events and crises.

Endemics involve the smallest scale of viral infection. An endemic is a kind of disease that caters to a specific area, community, or region. However, its distinguishing factor is the fact that this disease serves as a constant presence in that community due to various environmental factors. For example, malaria is endemic to various places in Africa. Dengue fever is endemic throughout Southeast Asia. Endemics are usually not a huge cause for concern until they are elevated to a status of an outbreak.

An outbreak is something that, unlike endemics, doesn't stay exclusive to a particular area or region. For example, in 2019 there was an outbreak of dengue fever in Hawaii. However, dengue is known to only be endemic to Africa, Southeast Asia, and South America. The fact that it was able to spread throughout Hawaii, an area that dengue is not endemic to, was enough to be classified as an outbreak. Typically, outbreaks are distinguished from endemic infections based on the expectedness of a disease. If a particular spread of disease is expected in that region, then it is endemic. If a disease is spreading at an unexpected rate or in non-typical areas, then it can be classified as an outbreak.

Consider an epidemic to be an elevated outbreak. Usually, a disease is considered to be an epidemic when it is actively infecting more and more people to a point where it becomes difficult to control the spread. Usually, an epidemic is a disease that is vastly growing - in terms of number of infected people - but remains exclusive to a single area or country. However, when an epidemic is able to cross borders and manifest itself in other countries, that is when it becomes classified as a pandemic.

When a pandemic takes place, conditions are at their gravest. An epidemic shows that there is a significant lapse on the part of a country or region to control the spread of a disease. A pandemic is proof that the whole world is not immune and the mobilization efforts of dealing with the disease become a lot more complex. There have been many pandemics throughout the course of human history. Some of them have proven to be more calamitous than others, but more on that later.

Why Do Pandemics Keep Happening?

It seems almost counterintuitive for a pandemic to occur now, doesn't it? Given that we are a thriving and resilient species, you would think that we would have solved the problem of pandemics by now. Unfortunately, we still have a lot to learn about them. Developments in the field of health and medicine have better equipped the human civilization for dealing with outbreaks of disease and illnesses. Despite this progress, we are still not able to completely eliminate the spread of infectious diseases altogether.

By exposing yourself to the contents of this book, you will gain further insights into how pandemics happen and what lapses took place that allowed for diseases to spread. Disease transmission is enabled by certain mistakes that human beings might make. The spread of infectious disease, like many other life-threatening situations, is not a problem without a solution. There are some very clear principles and mechanisms in place that are proven to work in fighting the spread of disease. And yet, in spite of that, pandemics continue to wreak havoc on the world every so often.

Containing the spread of disease is not as easy as one may assume. It requires the collective effort of various people spanning various races, nations, social classes, and industries. Similar to issues such as global warming or income inequality, the solutions to pandemic can't be brought about or executed by just one person. It's not just a select group of people who huddle up inside a conference room and produce a one-size-fits-all kind of solution that is meant to save all of mankind. Sadly, that's just not how problem-solving works when it comes to global issues.

Hopefully by the end of this book, you will have gained further insight into why pandemics happen and why human beings are falling short in the prevention of pandemics in the first place. In order to really prevent the occurrences of future pandemics, it's going to require the concerted effort of a critical mass of people. All of that starts with information gathering and knowledge sharing. This is why books such as this are very important. They help provide added perspective and guidance on dealing with crises that bring about a lot of fear and irrational behavior.

Why is It Important to Prepare for the Next Pandemic?

There are many things that continually threaten human existence on a daily basis. Global warming has been a serious threat for quite some time now. Nuclear war is also a continuing possibility with rising geopolitical tensions. However, there is something that is so uniquely dangerous about the emergence of a pandemic. Unlike global warming, its spread and destruction are going to be incredibly fast and dramatic. Unlike nuclear war, the threat of a pandemic is not always so easily controllable. Of course, that isn't to undermine the gravity and seriousness of these other threats. Rather, it's just important to stress that pandemics are also serious threats that really deserve just as much attention and concern on the part of the general public.

This is why it's essential to read up on literary resources such as this book. It's important to orient yourself with various scholarly resources to make sure that you always know what to do to prepare for such a serious threat. If people let their guard down by not taking such a threat seriously, it could spell potential doom for a large chunk of the population. This book isn't going to be the answer to the problems brought about by a pandemic. However, it is a contribution to the overall solution - one that everyone needs to play a part in if it is to succeed.

So far, we've been falling asleep at the wheel. We've been in the middle of one big nap. Dozens of pandemics have come and gone, and we have very little to show for it with regards to our preparedness and capacity to deal. It's time for the human race to wake up from this nap and start fighting back. Infectious diseases are no laughing matter. They are very serious issues that require our real attention as a civilization. It would be very foolish to just wait for the day when things get too bad to the point that we are no longer capable of rolling with the punches.

The day that human beings stop taking external threats seriously is the day that they no longer think it important to adapt to the world around them. And, as Darwin so eloquently put it, those who fail to adapt fail to survive.

Chapter 1:

A Brief History of Pandemics

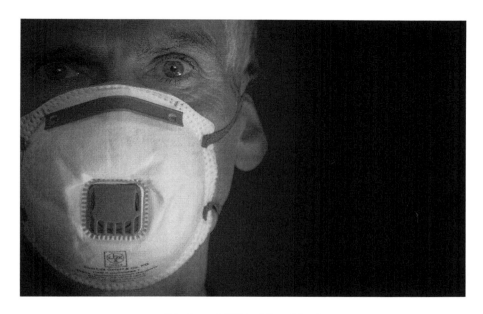

Black and White Face Mask

One of the greatest feats of the human species was the invention of mechanisms that allow travel across the land, sea, and air. However, one of the caveats of human beings now being scattered all around the world is the enabling of the spread of disease. We have faced numerous pandemics throughout the history of civilization and are currently in the midst of dealing with the COVID-19 pandemic. It's important for us to learn from the past to better address both current and future pandemics. Where did we go right? What did we do wrong? What can be improved upon?

In order for us to come up with the answers to these questions, we have to take a stroll down memory lane and try to uncover the narratives behind history's pandemics. Historians always say that the best ways for us to figure out the mysteries of the present is to look to the past.

Some of the World's Most Devastating Pandemics

Bubonic Plague (1347 - 1351) Death Toll: 200 Million

The Bubonic plague or *Black Death* that ravaged various parts of Europe, Asia, and Africa in the mid-1300s is considered by many to be the single most devastating pandemic to have ever threatened mankind. The general belief is that the plague originated in Asia and jumped to neighboring continents via rats who were serving as hosts to the fleas which were carrying the disease. These rats were able to make it from country to country by living on merchant ships which were used for trade among countries. The disease was caused by a strain of the *Yersinia pestis* bacterium which is believed to now be extinct. The plague spread to the point that most of Europe had to resort to discarding corpses in mass graves.

Smallpox (1520) Death Toll: 56 Million

The smallpox disease that originated in 1520 was so devastating that it was estimated to have reduced the population of a densely populated Aztec city by 40% in a single year. The disease is also known to have contributed to the easy colonization of these ancient civilizations by Spanish conquerors. On top of that, the disease was able to make its way over the Atlantic as well during the 1700s when trade and travel between America and Europe became more rampant. In Europe, it was estimated that around 60 million people had died from smallpox during the 18th century. Fortunately, the disease has now been curbed and a vaccine has already been developed to immunize people against the disease.

Spanish Flu (1918 - 1919) Death Toll: 40 to 50 Million

It was estimated that around half a billion people were infected by the Spanish Flu back in the early 1900s in the middle of World War 1. Of that half billion, around 40 to 50 million succumbed to the disease. The spread of the flu was made a lot easier due to the first World War. Soldiers and other participants of the war were often exposed to the harshest and most unhygienic conditions during that time. Also, they were often huddled up and cramped in incredibly close quarters. This made it much easier for the virus to jump from one host to another. On top of that, people weren't necessarily practicing the best nutritional habits as a result of the war. This led to a compromised immune system and a higher exposure to the virus.

Asian Flu (1957 - 1958) Death Toll: One Million

The next big influenza virus to take the world stage after the Spanish Flu was the Asian Flu (H2N2) which originated in China. The virus was deemed to have been a blend of different avian flu viruses. Experts would say that the virus was developed as a result of various animal wildlife being kept in close quarters with very minimal sanitation protocols. The disease would later go on to kill more than one million people. Even though the flu originated in China, it managed to infect people in Singapore, Hong Kong, and even some coastal cities of the United States.

Hong Kong Flu (1968 - 1970) Death Toll: One Million

Once the world had managed to recover from the Asian Flu, another major influenza would emerge just a decade later. Influenza A(H3N2) is actually a virus that is descended from the H2N2 virus via an antigenic shift. Essentially, the original virus that caused the Asian Flu mutated and formed another virus which would eventually come to be known as the Hong Kong Flu. It first originated in Hong Kong the summer of 1968. By the end of the year, the flu had managed to travel to Vietnam, Singapore, Philippines, Australia, and Europe. Soldiers returning to the States from the Vietnam war were also known to have carried the disease to America as well. In spite of the lethality of the Asian Flu in China a decade prior, very little changes or preparations were made to handle outbreaks. As such, the Hong Kong Flu managed to take the lives of more than one million people.

HIV/AIDS (1981 - present) Death Toll: 25 to 35 Million

Unlike the other recent pandemics in modern history, the HIV/AIDS pandemic is not one that was caused by an influenza virus. However, the handling of the HIV virus has shown the general lack of sophistication in the management of infectious diseases on a global scale. Since the virus was first discovered in 1981, it has been documented to have killed more than 35 million people. It was known to have originated in Africa via a chimpanzee virus that transferred to humans. There is currently no cure for HIV, but there are certain medications which allow HIV patients to experience a regular life span as long as they undergo regular treatment.

SARS (2002 - 2003) Death Toll: 770

SARS or Severe Acute Respiratory Syndrome is a very fatal and contagious respiratory illness. It was first discovered in China back in late 2002. During that time, China was a hotbed for trade and tourism, which led to many people unknowingly carrying the SARS virus back to their home countries. However, while the SARS virus could indeed be fatal, it managed to only leave a death toll of 770 people. This is not an insignificant number by any means, but it is much lower than the deaths caused by other flu-based pandemics throughout history.

Swine Flu (2009 - 2010) Death Toll: 200 Thousand

The Swine Flu or H1N1 pandemic was deemed to have originated in Mexico in the 2nd quarter of 2009. However, the strength and spread of the virus was so significant that it had managed to infect almost 1.5 billion people around the world within a span of a year. Certain estimates place the total number of deaths at around 200 thousand people conservatively. However, numerous reports also suggest that more than half a million people perished as a result of the H1N1 virus. As the disease was spreading, it was deemed to only have major effects on kids and young adults. With this particular virus, it seemed like older people had developed a natural immunity and tolerance for the disease. Today a vaccine for the H1N1 virus is readily available for use by the mass public.

MERS (2012 - present) Death Toll: 850

The MERS virus or Middle East Respiratory Syndrome coronavirus was first reported in Saudi Arabia. All of the documented cases so far have been linked to people who have either resided in or traveled to the Arabian Peninsula. The symptoms associated with the disease mostly revolve around respiratory illnesses like pneumonia. There is currently no vaccine or cure for the virus, but it hasn't been known to have as massive a spread or fatality rate as the H1N1 virus. There are many opposing claims to the origins of the disease. However, the virus has been known to be found in camels and bats.

COVID-19 (2019 - present) Death Toll: 122 Thousand

As this is being written, the COVID-19 coronavirus has cemented itself to be one of the gravest pandemics in modern history. The whole

COVID-19 pandemic is currently considered a very serious public health issue. Coronaviruses compose a typically large family of viruses that are found in all sorts of animals all over the world. Sometimes, these coronaviruses in animals can spread and infect people as well, as evidenced by the MERS and SARS viruses. The new COVID-19 virus is just another variation of that kind of disease.

It was known to have originated in the wet markets of Wuhan, China. In these markets, different animals like bats, chickens, and seafood are cramped in closed and unsanitary spaces. This has led these wet markets to be breeding grounds for germs and disease. Ultimately, the COVID-19 disease managed to spread out all over the world and has killed around 122,000 people to date.

Was It God's Wrath?

In the old days, people didn't necessarily have as sophisticated an understanding of science as we do now. In fact, most of what was deemed unexplainable or overly complex in the past was often chalked up to be some kind of divine act or intervention. Whenever diseases would spread and outbreaks would take place, people would often just attribute it to the gods punishing people for their sins and misdeeds. Instead of looking at it from a medical and scientific perspective, people saw the situation more as the manifestation of the wrath of the gods. Naturally, as you might expect, an unscientific approach to solving outbreaks isn't going to be the most effective one. This kind of mindset led to the deaths of millions of people, especially during the bubonic plague.

Hindsight is always 20/20, as the cliché goes. We know that it was the propagation of trade and commerce that allowed for the spread of disease. However, during those times, people often saw outbreaks as an opportunity to smear incumbent governments or leadership. It was easy to use any outbreaks of disease as an excuse to overthrow a government by merely saying that the gods had not been pleased with their style of leadership. It was an accepted belief that plagues of disease were cast upon the people for the actions of their leaders. Obviously, none of these claims were founded in science and they did nothing to absolve the situation whatsoever.

Nowadays, the human race has evolved to become more sophisticated in its relationship to science and medicine. We now understand that diseases are typically caused by germs, bacteria, and viruses. Of course, this developed understanding of disease has led to us having better responses and mechanisms in place to counteract the spread of infectious diseases. However, that doesn't mean that we have perfected our disease response protocols. There is still far too much to learn about how society can better improve its protocols for dealing with the spreads of disease.

The Globalization of Disease

One of the most effective and efficient disease containment protocols was invented during the bubonic plague of the 14th century. In fact, it was deemed to be so effective that it continues to be a protocol that is widely practiced today. When the bubonic plague was becoming increasingly rampant in Europe, Italy decided to act fast and protect their cities by closing entry to their ports in Venice. Any ships that were arriving in Venetian ports were required to anchor their vessels and stay for a period of 40 days before disembarking. In Italian, 40 days roughly translates to *quaranta giorni*. From that, the idea of *quarantine* was born. Fast forward a few hundred years later and the practice of quarantining has become one of the most valuable tools in the medical industry for containing the spread of disease.

A few centuries after the devastating bubonic plague, the cholera outbreak in the 19th century prompted health and medical professionals to turn to geography and statistical analysis to combat the spread of disease. A doctor named John Snow discovered in 1854 that the cholera outbreak was being further enabled by means of tainted water. He determined through geographical and statistical analysis that people were contracting cholera from their shared water sources. He indicated the mortality of various neighborhoods in map form to inform the general public of the spread of the disease.

These days, there are now more sophisticated means of documenting and analyzing the spread of a disease. After the MERS disease created an outbreak in South Korea in 2015, the country became incredibly traumatized by the event. Immediately after the outbreak the government, together with the country's top medical institutions, developed various protocols to further enhance their disease containment protocols in case a new outbreak took place. When the COVID-19 virus spread to South Korea in the earlier parts of 2020, the entire country was quick to roll out mass testing kits to make sure that all of their citizens had access to tests. An intricate contact-tracing system was also implemented through the use of surveillance systems and mobile data gathering. This way, it was easier for the government to track the movements of any patients who might have been infected or exposed to the virus. The system, while considered to be quite advanced relative to the rest of the world, is still far from perfect and shows some potential points of improvement.

Tracking the Spread of a Disease

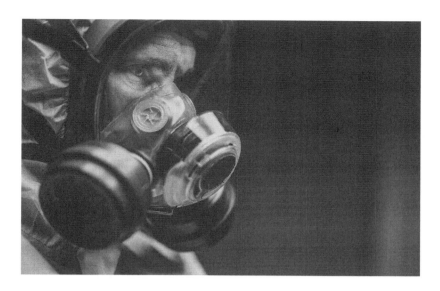

Mask and Hazmat Suit

It is important that diseases are assessed to determine how serious they are. With limited medical resources, it's essential that medical professionals are able to aggregate their time properly and prioritize diseases that are more dangerous and infectious. To do so, scientists have developed a basic unit of measurement to track the level of infectiousness of a particular disease. They called this measurement the Ro or the R *naught*. The number on the R *naught* is essentially a calculated estimate of how many people are bound to get infected by a person depending on the disease.

For example, the disease with the highest R *naught* rating is measles as it falls within the range of 12 to 18. This means that a person with measles is predicted to infect at least 12 to 18 people on average. Of course, these numbers can plummet depending on the level of vaccination that has taken place in a given population sample.

In modern history, measles isn't known to be one of the most dangerous diseases out there. It has a high R *naught* rating, but its spread has been dramatically curbed as a result of mass vaccination efforts along with developed immunity of certain communities.

Naturally, the more people there are who are immune to a particular disease, the less likely it will be for that disease to thrive. This is why vaccinations are very important in the fight against infectious diseases.

Currently, there is no generally agreed upon valuation of COVID-19's R *naught* rating within the scientific community. This is often attributed to the fact that various research efforts are still taking place with regards to this relatively new form of coronavirus.

The Pitfalls of Urbanization

If you take a look at all of the modern pandemics brought about by influenzas, it's hard not to see the similarities with the pandemics of earlier history. It seems as if we still haven't learned from our old mistakes and are continually enabling the spread of disease right now. There are more sophisticated mechanisms and protocols that are in place now to combat the spread of disease. However, these protocols are far from being enough. The prime instigator of the spread of infectious diseases is the fact that we now live in a highly urbanized global community. Interactions between people who live in different parts of the world are much easier now than they ever have been. Humanity has developed a certain level of dependence on neighboring tribes, countries, and cultures. This has paved the way for substantial economic and social development, but it has also enabled the spread of infectious disease.

On top of that, urbanization is fueling an already alarming density problem in developing nations. As urban cities become bigger and more expensive to live in, rural residents are driven to reside in cramped and dense neighborhoods. It's living conditions such as this that can drive the spread of disease. On top of that, proper health care isn't a luxury that is readily accessible to those who don't come from higher economic classes. In addition to living in cramped and dense neighborhoods, people of lower economic classes tend to have poorer health and immune systems as well. These make them all the more susceptible and vulnerable to the contraction of infectious diseases. Commercial air travel is also becoming a lot cheaper and more accessible to people. Naturally, this kind of connectedness between people and places can make it easy for disease to jump from one community to another.

Chapter 2:

Problems With Preparation

If you purely assess the previous chapter on its own merits and with no additional context, it would be easy to assume that we have come a long way. Obviously, nothing like the bubonic plague has ever taken place ever since it came around in the 14th century. The world hasn't had to deal with a disease that has rapidly infected and killed as many people in a short amount of time like the bubonic plague did. In fact, if you take a look at the history of pandemics in the previous chapter again, you will see that the emergence of each disease is killing fewer and fewer people as time goes on. From that perspective alone, you might be able to gather that the world is just gradually getting better at minimizing the destructive effects of these diseases with each passing day. And it's true that every day people are becoming less and less likely to die from some kind of rapidly accelerating infectious disease.

There is some definite good news about how we handle pandemics; there is some cause for joy. However, it is not a cause for complacency. In fact, there are still plenty of things to be concerned about. With the emergence of the COVID-19 pandemic, the world is reminded that infectious diseases are still very much present day dangers to modern society. Also, if you take a look at the highlights of the previous chapter again, you will find that there are more new emerging infectious diseases nowadays then there ever have been. The pandemics of the past were definitely more destructive, but it's easier for outbreaks to take place today and they're becoming more rampant. The amount of annual outbreaks that take place in the world have already tripled since 1980. Even when you take a look at just the infectious diseases from the past couple decades, SARS, MERS, and COVID-19 all took place within a small time window. The MERS and

COVID-19 viruses are even overlapping now. From that perspective, you could say the world is more vulnerable now than it has ever been to infectious diseases. We are better able to deal with infectious diseases now, but we are also more exposed to them than ever before.

More People. More Problems.

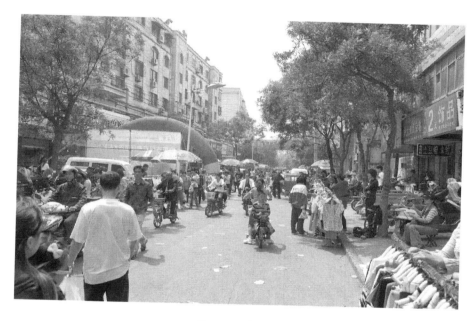

Overpopulation

One of the most obvious reasons that infectious diseases are much more dangerous now than they have ever been is the fact that there are more people nowadays to infect. In the span of just 50 years, the total number of people in the world has more than doubled from just a little under 3.6 billion to nearly eight billion people now. Keep in mind that viruses and infectious diseases only thrive when they are able to latch themselves onto hosts. When there are more people, diseases have more potential hosts that allow them to grow and prosper. Whenever there is an outbreak of disease, these viruses are able to survive when they prey on an unsuspecting host. And these days, an unsuspecting host might be exposed to twice as many people as they would have been back in the 1970s. This is especially true in the world's most densely populated cities.

The amount of livestock in the world has also increased as the human population has grown. Remember that a lot of these viruses that fuel pandemics typically come from animals. The demand for livestock is so great now that the animal farming industry is at an all-time high. According to data published in a BBC article, there is more livestock now in the world than has existed in the past 10,000 years leading up to 1960 combined (Walsh, 2020). Think about that. As people continually expose themselves to animals who are forced to live in such unsanitary cramped conditions, the threat of infectious disease becomes more prevalent.

An Economic Growth Paradox

COVID-19 is a very powerful case study in how the world economy is largely to blame when it comes to the strength and spread of infectious diseases. When you take a look at the global economy now, everything is so easily accessible. Everything is more connected now than it has ever been. Mass production, shipping, and supply are all the rage in big business these days. Ironically enough, this large-scale global economy with its increasingly complex supply chains is also very much vulnerable to the monsters that it creates. As COVID-19 has demonstrated, when a pandemic gets strong enough, the world has to shut down significantly in order to address public health issues. This has led to the plummeting of stock markets all around the world. In fact, many pundits say that the world is on the brink of a global depression if the pandemic isn't resolved soon enough. The global economy is holding on for dear life, but it's also largely to blame for its own suffering.

Think about how easy it is for a disease-causing virus to get from one spot of the world to another in a matter of just a few hours. In the past, when viruses would cling onto shipment packages or luggage, they would easily die out over the course of a transatlantic voyage. However, that's not the case these days. Everything is just so fast. It's the reason that the economy is growing at such a rapid rate. It's so easy to get items from Point A to Point B in just a matter of hours. With that, a virus is able to hold on to its strength and vitality long enough to wait for a viable host to be exposed to them once more between the delivery and receipt of a shipment. It's true that the human race has made some very significant advances in the fight against infectious disease. The medical community nowadays has a lot to show for itself. However, there is also no denying the fact that our growth as a species has also led us to become much more vulnerable to these scary threats that evolve at a much faster rate than human beings do.

Institutional Lapses

When penicillin was first discovered in 1928, it was considered to be a revolutionary breakthrough. The discovery of penicillin led to the development of antibiotics that would go on to save hundreds of millions of lives over the decades. However, experts have discovered that emerging bacteria is also developing more resistance towards these drugs with each passing year. This is why infectious diseases persist as one of the most significant threats to humanity even today. It's not just the fact that there are more people to infect. It's also the fact that these viruses are evolving, mutating, and getting stronger themselves. So, while the human race is busy trying to fortify its defenses, the enemy is doing the exact same thing. According to a report published by the CDC, almost three million infections that took place in the United States in 2019 were caused by antibiotic-resistant pathogens. Of the million people who were infected, an estimated 35,000 of them died (Healio, 2019). That's approximately one death to an antibiotic-resistant pathogen every 15 minutes in the United States alone. As these diseases are getting stronger and growing more resistant to the advances in medicine, it wouldn't be too farfetched to think that even everyday illnesses could prove to be fatal to us in the future if we fail to act and progress in our treatment protocols.

In 2013, the World Bank released a hypothetical estimate of how much the global economy would have to pay if the 1918 Spanish flu took place in 2013. The number that they came up with was around four trillion dollars. To put things into perspective, that's higher than the total individual GDPs of economic powerhouse countries like Germany, India, the United Kingdom, and France. If you take a look at the economic damages that COVID-19 is causing so far, it can be hard to come up with definite quantitative measurements of how much money the world is really losing. However, it's plainly obvious that the world is currently suffering and that the global economy is caught in a crippled state.

In spite of that hypothetical simulation that was drawn up by the World Bank, there have been no significant advances or reforms put in place by the world's leading economies to combat an influenza pandemic like the one from 1918. Even when you look at an esteemed institution like the World Health Organization, it's not too hard to see where they failed and where they could have improved. The way that the WHO handled SARS was quite commendable. However, its response to the more recent outbreaks like Swine Flu, MERS, and now COVID-19 is much less impressive. In fact, there are plenty of calls on social media forums and platforms that are currently advocating for a complete overhaul of the WHO structure. There is a growing general sentiment of dissatisfaction and distrust with how the WHO has handled these deadly pandemics as of late.

The Antivaxxers

At its core, even individual human psychology is to blame for the propagation of infectious diseases. If you've been paying enough attention to the news recently, you will know that there is a formidable mass of people out there who are advocating that vaccines be boycotted. Typically, a claim such as this should be dismissed immediately, especially when they are not founded on principles of science and profound empiricism. However, with the propagation of fake news, mass hysteria has ensued and more people are not having themselves or their kids vaccinated. This false information surrounding the make-believe dangers of vaccination has forced the WHO's hand in naming the "antivaxxer" movement as one of the world's gravest public health threats. In fact, in various places around the world, the long-dead measles disease has made a resurrection as a result of this clout surrounding vaccination.

The Current Problem

COVID-19 is the latest pandemic to ravage the world and it has done so on a dramatically significant scale. It found its origins in a very densely populated city in China, which is one of the most economically connected and prosperous nations in the world. It is possible that China's poor political acts of neglect and willful silencing led to the spread of the disease all over the world. However, that is a political debate for another time. The fact of the matter is that the disease originated there and that it wasn't contained. There were poor control efforts on the part of the Chinese authorities and that led to the eventual pandemic that it has become. Now that the disease has reached a pandemic scale, it's important to assess how the world and individual nations are responding.

Naturally, scientists are making use of the various technological tools that are at their disposal in order to combat the spread of the disease. This is why so much information surrounding the biological makeup of the virus was made available so quickly. Medical advances have enabled us to identify what the virus looks like and why it's so lethal. Currently, there is no vaccine for the COVID-19 virus, but various research projects are underway in the development of such a vaccine. The unfortunate news here is that it will take quite some time before a vaccine is deemed safe for the market. It will have to undergo some very strict medical testing protocols before it gains approval for commercial production and supply. On that front, you can make the argument that the response to the virus is as sophisticated as it was before. The speed at which scientists and researchers were able to identify the makeup of the virus is unprecedented. On the other hand, there are many people who are getting sick and dying without the existence of a readily available vaccine.

When you take a look at the individual responses of human beings to the emergence of the virus, things get a little more interesting. On an institutional front, things are pretty advanced. Medical institutions are working round-the-clock to contain the spread of the disease. However, when you look at it on a more micro-scale, you might be able to say that our individual responses are rather medieval. We mentioned earlier in this book that the idea of quarantine was first established in the 14th century when the bubonic plague was at its peak. It's strange to think that seven centuries later, we would still be employing the same tactics that people of the past did. The way that you're locked up in your home now is fundamentally not much different than when voyagers were locked up in ships back in the 14th century. In terms of our responses, a lot of things are much more different and advanced now. And yet, a lot of things are still the same. Whether or not that's a good thing is up to you.

Chapter 3:

What Can We Do in the Midst of a

Pandemic?

One of the most complicated aspects of living in a pandemic is the uncertainty. Much like when a war takes place, there's just no telling how long the crisis is going to last. It's not like diseases and viruses will set deadlines for themselves. They aren't going to just instantly terminate their spread on predetermined dates. That's not how pandemics work. When people are stuck in one, they may freak out and act irrationally. Naturally, this is the absolute worst thing that you could do when you're stuck in a pandemic.

People in general aren't typically exposed to pandemics that affect them directly. So, when a pandemic starts garnering enough strength to the point where most people in the world start to really become affected, it creates the opportunity for chaos to ensue. That is the last thing we want to happen when a pandemic strikes. A pandemic in itself is already a very chaotic crisis. The only way to combat such a crisis would be through a community effort of systematic responses and science-backed solutions.

If you subscribe yourself to the category of people who are unsure about how you should be conducting yourself in the midst of a pandemic, then this chapter is definitely for you. This segment of the book is going to take a deep dive into everything that you need to be doing as an individual when you're caught in a pandemic. Again, overcoming a pandemic isn't just a matter of waiting around for the powers that be to come up with an umbrella solution for everyone. There are some very specific duties and responsibilities that you need to fulfill in your own individual capacity to help alleviate the spread and destruction of an infectious disease.

More than anything, you have to understand that while a pandemic is a serious issue, there isn't any need for you to panic. Again, as has been evidenced in previous chapters, a pandemic doesn't necessarily imply the end of the world. The human race has always managed to survive past pandemics. There is no reason why a current one should be any different. It's just a matter of you making sure that you know what to do to best protect yourself and ensure your own personal safety during such scary and troublesome times.

With that, if you are ever feeling like you aren't sure of what it is you need to be doing, then just make sure that you browse through the items and concepts listed here. Again, there's no need to devolve into a state of panic and chaotic behavior. Maintain your composure and try to keep a level head. Allow your reason and better judgement to come through. The most optimal way to make it through a crisis like a pandemic would be to always engage in best practices.

Social Distancing

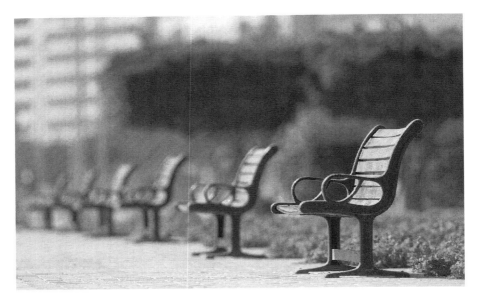

Social Distancing

Even when the spread of an infectious disease is still in the stage of an outbreak, you might already hear the term *social distancing* get thrown out there. When the spread of a disease gets serious enough to the point where it becomes a pandemic, you're still going to be bombarded with advisories and implementations on social distancing. One might come to the summation that social distancing is a tool to address the spread of a pandemic. However, the whole concept of social distancing might not necessarily be so obvious to most people. And in order for such a measure to work properly, it's essential that a critical mass of people really get behind the movement by fully understanding why it works and why it's important.

What is Social Distancing?

To put it simply, social distancing is the act of establishing a physical distance between yourself and another human being. However, the Center for Disease Control and Prevention (CDC) have a set of parameters that truly constitute systemic social distancing. According to the CDC, to practice proper social distancing, one must always do the following:

- Maintain a distance of at least six feet or two meters between yourself and other people
- Avoid going to places where there are large crowds or mass gatherings
- Stay at home and avoid going out unless it's absolutely essential to do so

Sometimes, when a pandemic gets particularly serious, some governments will resort to enforcing lockdowns or community quarantines in certain places in response to the CDC's call for social distancing. The policies and regulations can differ depending on the governing institution. In such lockdowns, people are usually encouraged to stay at home at all times. There are some exceptions to the rule in order to make sure that society's general needs are being met. Typically, when a lockdown is being enforced, non-essential businesses and offices might have to close down to force their workers and customers to stay home. Although, during a pandemic, there are certain businesses and establishments that need to stay open. There are also some people who are considered to be essential personnel during a pandemic and still have to report to work in order to keep society afloat. These people can include doctors, nurses, medical technicians, janitors, policemen, firemen, garbage collectors, food suppliers and manufacturers, etc. In a pandemic, these people are often referred to as the *frontliners*. However, when the nature of your job is considered non-essential during a pandemic, you are advised to stay at home and isolate yourself from the rest of the world.

Some countries might take a stricter approach to social distancing by instituting strict lockdowns with curfews, border checkpoints, patrolling officers, and punitive policies. On the other hand, there might be governments that will take a more lenient approach to promoting social distancing. Regardless, social distancing, while simple in principle, happens to be one of the most effective tools in combating the spread of a disease.

What Makes It Effective?

There are actually two layers to why social distancing is one of the most effective tools that you can use to combat the spread of the disease. On the first level, social distancing can help in flattening the curve. Next, social distancing can help in preventing the spread of the disease altogether. But before we get to that, let's talk about what it means to flatten the curve. You might already be familiar with the concept of flattening the curve in articles or videos that you've been exposed to on the internet, but you might not really grasp the ins and outs of it.

To put it simply, the *curve* that is being referred to here is a figure on a graph. This graph details the amount of people who are getting infected by the disease over an established period of time. When more and more people are getting infected during a pandemic within a short span of time, the curve on the graph becomes more pronounced. To *flatten the curve* merely means to spread out the rate of infection among people across a longer span of time. This way, hospitals and medical professionals aren't overwhelmed by the severity of the crisis. This makes them better equipped to deal with people infected by the virus as they come. When that curve flattens out, the containment and treatment of a virus becomes a lot more feasible and manageable.

Next, there is the matter of slowing down the spread of the disease or even the possibility of stopping it altogether. You have to keep in mind that a disease is only made infectious due to a virus or bacteria. However, these viruses are usually incapable of surviving on their own for prolonged periods of time. In order for them to survive and multiply, they must latch themselves onto hosts who haven't developed immunity against them. This is why when there is an outbreak of a new disease, a lot of people tend to get sick quickly because there is no established immunity in human beings just yet. However, by practicing social distancing, people aren't giving these viruses a chance to jump from one host to another so easily. With that, it makes it more difficult for the virus to spread around and even survive. This is precisely why social distancing is a very important practice whenever there is a pandemic going on.

Staying Updated and Informed

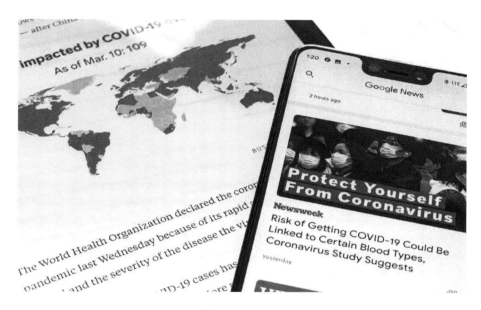

News Articles

Another very important thing to do while in a pandemic is to constantly stay updated and informed. If you are reading a book like this, then that's already a good sign. It means that you are doing your part to keep yourself informed on the science and history behind pandemics. However, more than that, it's very important that you also keep yourself updated on the many things that are going on around you.

One of the biggest pitfalls in the age of information is the massive spread and popularity of false news. Sometimes, in an effort to incite hysteria and hype, people might spread around false information. This can be very dangerous, especially in the middle of a pandemic. People must always be fed correct and true information so that they have the necessary tools to arm themselves against a virus and disease. On your part, you have to make sure that you are only taking your news from reputable institutions and sources. During a pandemic, you can always rely on organizations like the Center for Disease Control and Prevention along with the World Health Organization. Be sure to also stay updated on the recommendations and policies set forth by your government officials. Addressing a pandemic is going to require mass cooperation. To know your responsibilities as a citizen, you have to catch yourself up on whatever policies are being enforced in your area.

Self-Quarantine

Ultimately, if you are non-essential personnel in times of a pandemic, the absolute best thing that you can do is to just stay home and quarantine yourself. Granted, this is not the easiest and most natural thing for human beings to do these days. Of course, we currently live in a world where everything is designed to be mobile. It's an everyday occurrence for most of us to wake up in the morning, get dressed, and then leave the house in order to be productive. However, that is not something that would be advisable in times of a pandemic.

Again, it's very important that the general public adhere to the principles of social distancing. Understandably, there will be a lot of resistance and hesitation on the part of ordinary individuals, but this is still the best course of action for people to take. If you feel like you're uninformed of the common principles and best practices behind putting yourself into quarantine, then that's okay. Pandemics usually present unprecedented times, so it's normal for people to not know what to do. When you put yourself into quarantine or lockdown, here are a few things that you might want to keep in mind.

Working from Home

If you are lucky enough to have a career that still affords you the opportunity to be productive even while you're on quarantine, then capitalize on that. Yes, these are very scary times. But you don't want to exacerbate those fears even further by not knowing whether you will have any source of income or not. So, if you are able to work from home, then try to continue to do so. For one, you still need your income in order to support yourself and your lifestyle in the midst of this pandemic. Also, it's very important that you stay productive while you're in quarantine.

If possible, set up a workstation in your house that is purely dedicated to your work. It can be tempting to just lie down in bed all day and work on your laptop. However, you have to learn to separate your work from your home life. Associate your bed with sleeping and relaxing, and try to avoid doing any work there. Also, if possible, try dressing up as if you were really going to work. This is going to help place you in a mindset of productivity even while you're just at home.

If you don't have a job that affords you the opportunity of working at home, then it's possible that you will feel anxious about your source of income. First, it's important that you brush yourself up on whatever support your government would be able to provide you (more on that later). You still want to fulfill your responsibilities in making sure that you have a steady source of income. If possible, try checking online to see if you can monetize any of your skills. These days, it can be easy to get a job on the internet for just about anything so as long as you have some talent or proficiency in a particular skill. Try to do whatever you can to ensure that you still have a revenue stream even during a pandemic.

Stocking Up on Necessities

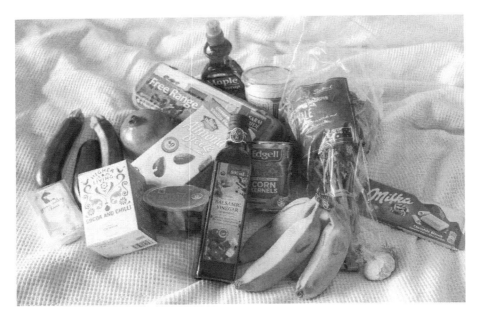

Groceries

Of course, you still have to stock up on necessities even when you're on quarantine. However, the key to making social distancing work is if you avoid leaving your home as much as possible. Try to avoid going to any public places unless it's for the acquisition of certain necessities or if you have an emergency situation. Naturally, you should still be allowed to go to the supermarket or grocery stores to stock up on goods for your home, but you should try to minimize your shopping trips to limit your possible exposure to the disease. When you go shopping, try to buy in reasonable bulk. You don't want to hoard to the point that you're leaving nothing for others, but you should try to buy a reasonable amount so that you don't have to pay another visit to the store anytime soon. Here is a general list of things that you want to stock up on while you're quarantined:

Toiletries and Hygiene

- common medications like pain relievers, electrolytes, cough medicine, etc.
- toilet paper
- hand soap, hand sanitizer, and rubbing alcohol
- body soap and shampoos
- facial care items
- house cleaning materials
- dishwashing liquid or soap
- laundry detergent
- feminine hygiene products, etc.

Food

- Dried beans and legumes
- whole wheat and grains
- canned soup
- protein powders
- dried fruits
- nuts
- cured meats
- cooking oil
- spices
- frozen meats and poultry
- eggs
- drinking water
- pet food, etc.

Receiving Government Support or Welfare

Don't be afraid to accept government support or welfare when a pandemic is going on. You are entitled to such services if you are a taxpayer. Try to update yourself on whatever relief efforts your government might be providing. No matter how small or insignificant it may seem, you have to maximize your opportunities in a time of crisis. If you are incapable of working, then try to ask your local governments if there are any temporary employment opportunities or unemployment benefits they can offer you while a quarantine is being enforced.

Developing New Skills

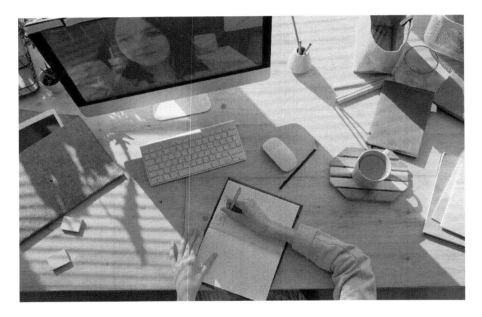

Working on Desk

Lastly, you are going to have a lot of extra time when you're just going to be stuck at home. During this time, it's important that you still stay productive by getting something done whenever you can. If possible, try learning or developing new skills for yourself. For example, you can teach yourself to play a musical instrument or read more books. It's also good if you try developing skills that you can potentially monetize for an extra source of income. For instance, you can try to practice baking. Then, you can sell your baked goods within your community to try to earn an extra buck. There are so many things that you can do with the extra time. It's important that you try to make the most of it all.

Chapter 4:

What Should We Do Moving

Forward?

As you may have come to expect, it's not enough that we know what to do now as the world is currently enveloped in a crisis. It's just as important to know about what the next steps should be to make sure that we are better prepared for the next one. Knowing how to act in the middle of a crisis is very important, but it's always much better to be proactive when it comes to situations like these. As they keep on saying in the medical community, prevention is much better than cure. For the most part, most of the changes have to be institutional in nature. The world is just far too vast and complex nowadays. Any change or reform that takes place must be executed in a systematic manner. Otherwise, it wouldn't really have that much of an effect.

And on a more personal scale, individual preparedness is going to be key in addressing issues such as this as well. Again, there is a tendency to let primal human nature take over to the point of inciting mass hysteria when a crisis is ongoing. However, none of these hysterics are value-adding and must be avoided at all costs when there is a grave crisis going on. This is exactly where individual preparedness comes in. It always helps to know that you are protected by the strength of institutions and community, but it's a different kind of comfort when you are able to rely on yourself to survive the next big pandemic as well.

This chapter is going to touch on the important probable next steps for the whole world when it comes to preparing for the next pandemic. Reforms and changes must be made. And these preparations must both be systematic and individualistic in nature. Ultimately, there is still a lot to be done in order to fully prepare ourselves for the next major health crisis.

Institutional Funding and Support

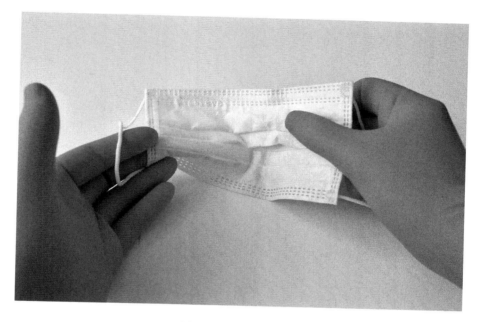

Gloves and Face Mask

It's already a complete metaphysical certainty that the next big virus is going to hit us again. None of us know when and none of us know how strong it's going to be. However, when we have a stronger system of protocols pertaining to global health, we will be in much better positions to handle it better. For one, we should strengthen our protocols in catching and identifying outbreaks quicker. The faster we are at responding to outbreaks, the easier they will be to contain.

Currently, the World Health Organization is the closest thing that we've got to a global watchdog when it comes to public health matters. And unfortunately, the funding that the WHO receives is not nearly enough to fully protect and ensure the safety of the world's nearly eight billion inhabitants. All around the world, national governments are favoring budget allocations for military and tourism over healthcare. This does not bode well for healthcare professionals whenever pandemics take place and the rest of the world has to shut down while they work.

More than just institutional changes, there is also a need to double our efforts on the development of vaccines. It was mentioned earlier that more diseases are growing increasingly resistant to emerging treatments and antibiotics. This means that one of the most effective ways to deal with diseases is to avoid getting sick in the first place. The development protocols of vaccines are incredibly complex and comprehensive, as they should be. However, it should also be taken into consideration that response time matters gravely in the event of an outbreak. More funding should be pooled into researching how we can best optimize and streamline the development of vaccines in times of an outbreak.

It all boils down to allocating funds for general preparedness. Every year, governments all over the world pour trillions into their military budgets. They justify it by saying that fortifying their military forces means a higher level of safety and protection for their citizens. Naturally, there is a point to be made there. However, the same argument can also be made for healthcare. When it comes to safety and protection against outbreaks of disease, it's the healthcare professionals who serve on the frontlines, not military personnel. Yes, there are constant military threats that plague various governments around the world. But as we have already established, there are just as many health threats that know no sovereignties or jurisdictions - and they are far more unforgiving.

Government Regulation on Sanitation

The improvement of public sanitation in commercial spaces is also a vital aspect of disease prevention. It's no secret that the influenzas that have incited the world's recent pandemics are a result of poor environmental conditions and sanitation practices in populated marketplaces. The swine flu virus which originated in Mexico was deemed to have come from wet markets that were selling different kinds of meats in unsanitary conditions. The same can be said of COVID-19 and the Asian Flu virus as well, except these came from wet markets that were located in China. There have got to be stricter government regulations on commercial institutions such as this with regards to their sanitary practices.

There is no reason for these kinds of marketplaces to exist when you take into consideration the kinds of risks that are involved. Sure, these kinds of marketplaces might be essential to a local economy. However, on a more global scale, when a pandemic strikes as a result of these unsanitary environments, the ends just don't justify the means anymore. The economic losses during a pandemic are much greater and much more difficult to recover from than just closing these unsanitary wet markets altogether.

And these strict government policies on sanitation shouldn't just be singling out wet markets either. The same principles on sanitation should also apply to mass public transportation and mass housing projects. The world is becoming more and more densely populated with each passing day. With that, it's important to ensure the health and safety of everyone by focusing on promoting proper sanitary practices in various public institutions.

Better Individual Preparedness

Lastly, it's very important that you prepare yourself for the next pandemic by doing this one simple thing: information gathering. The more you know, the better equipped you will be to arm yourself against these outbreaks and pandemics. Keep in mind that a well-informed community is a much stronger one.

Although a lot of the reforms and changes mainly concern the institutional levels, you can still do your part to properly handle a pandemic if you're in one and prepare for the next health crisis. Sometimes, this may involve increasing your own personal war chest and emergency savings to keep you afloat in case the economy comes to a standstill. You could also strive to live a healthier and fitter lifestyle to make sure that your immune system is performing at an optimal level. Or you may find yourself in a position to offer valuable advice and knowledge to the people around you about public health crises. Whatever the case, your individual effort still matters. Keep in mind that a mass accumulation of individual efforts can create a significant impact on society as a whole.

Conclusion

It may seem like the chaos that is being brought about by the prospect of pandemics has rendered the world to be a hopeless one to live in. It's very important that you eliminate that kind of mindset. Naturally, pandemics are disastrous situations and they definitely require your utmost concern and attention. Although, they are not a cause for you to lose hope. Again, it all goes back to human resilience. The proof is in the pudding. Our species would not have thrived and survived for as long as it has without being resilient. Hopefully this book will serve as fuel to the fire of resilience in the world. There have been many mistakes with regards to how we have handled pandemics, both past and present. However, these failures can also serve as a glimmer of hope moving forward to enable us to be better in how we conduct ourselves as a global community.

As individuals, there are so many things that we can do to prepare for the next big pandemic. We can read up on past pandemics and learn about the best practices along with the mistakes that we've made in history. It's also important that we make it a point to clamor for better funding for our medical institutions. Our health institutions and frontliners should always have easy access to the tools that they need to stay safe as they combat the spreads of disease. More funding should be pooled into research and development on vaccines to help keep us safe and sound. General preparedness is never something that you should be inclined to undermine or dismiss.

There are so many threats that the human race has to face on a day to day basis. And these threats encompass a variety of sectors, industries, and classes. They also come in varying levels of complexity and impact. But the human spirit should always remain steadfast and strong. At the end of the day, regardless of whatever obstacles we may come to face, human civilization must and will overcome. It's time for us to wake up from this nap that we've indulged in for quite some time now. It's time for us to lace up our gloves and fight back. It's time to get to work.

References

Centers for Disease Control and Prevention. (2020, February 11). *Social Distancing, Quarantine, and Isolation.* https://www.cdc.gov/coronavirus/2019-ncov/prevent-getting-sick/social-distancing.html

Healio. (2019, November 13). *CDC: Antibiotic resistance causes 1 death every 15 minutes* in US. https://www.healio.com/infectious-disease/antimicrobials/news/online/%7Bf30ac0ff-2016-47dc-8fd1-0cd729f0a3e8%7D/cdc-antibiotic-resistance-causes-1-death-every-15-minutes-in-us

Intermountain Healthcare. (2020, April 2). *What's the difference between a pandemic, an epidemic, endemic, and an outbreak?* https://intermountainhealthcare.org/blogs/topics/live-well/2020/04/whats-the-difference-between-a-pandemic-an-epidemic-endemic-and-an-outbreak/

Jarus, O. (2020, March 25). *20 of the worst epidemics and pandemics in history.* Live Science. https://www.livescience.com/worst-epidemics-and-pandemics-in-history.html

LePan, N. (2020, March 14). *Visualizing the History of Pandemics.* Visual Capitalist. https://www.visualcapitalist.com/history-of-pandemics-deadliest/

Walsh, B. (2020, March 25). *Covid-19: The history of pandemics.* BBC. https://www.bbc.com/future/article/20200325-covid-19-the-history-of-pandemics

Image Sources

Black and White Face Mask Pixabay (CC0). (n.d.):

https://pixabay.com/photos/mask-virus-pandemic-coronavirus-4934337/

Face Mask Pixabay (CC0). (n.d.):

https://pixabay.com/photos/virus-protection-coronavirus-woman-4898571/

Gloves and Face Mask Pixabay (CC0). (n.d.):

https://pixabay.com/photos/face-mask-covid-19-epidemic-4986596/

Groceries Unsplash (CC0). (n.d.): https://unsplash.com/photos/Hz4FAtKSLKo

Mask and Hazmat Suit Pixabay (CC0). (n.d.):

https://pixabay.com/photos/covid-19-coronavirus-dystopia-4987797/

News Articles Unsplash (CC0). (n.d.): https://unsplash.com/photos/qXfD_nG4j-U

Overpopulation Pixabay (CC0). (n.d.):

https://pixabay.com/photos/china-shopping-street-road-asia-728885/

Social Distancing Pixabay (CC0). (n.d.):

https://pixabay.com/photos/bench-seat-social-distance-park-5017748/

Viral Outbreak Pixabay (CC0). (n.d.):

https://pixabay.com/illustrations/covid-corona-coronavirus-virus-4948866/

Working on Desk Pexels (CC0). (n.d.):

https://www.pexels.com/photo/person-writing-on-notebook-4144923/

Printed in Great Britain
by Amazon